Fitness Tracker

I0421461

If you can measure it,

You can improve it.

WEEK 1

DATE:	WEIGHT:
HOW DO YOU FEEL?	
IF YOU CAN MEASURE IT, YOU CAN IMPROVE IT	

GOALS

1.
2.
3.

WORKOUT LOG

DATE:		WT.		CARDIO:				
	SET 1		SET 2		SET 3		SET 4	
EXERCISE	WT.	REP	WT.	REP	WT.	REP	WT.	REP

DATE:	WT.	CARDIO:

	SET 1		SET 2		SET 3		SET 4	
EXERCISE	WT.	REP	WT.	REP	WT.	REP	WT.	REP

DATE:		WT.		CARDIO:				
	SET 1		SET 2		SET 3		SET 4	
EXERCISE	WT.	REP	WT.	REP	WT.	REP	WT.	REP

DATE:		WT.		CARDIO:				
	SET 1		SET 2		SET 3		SET 4	
EXERCISE	WT.	REP	WT.	REP	WT.	REP	WT.	REP

DATE:		WT.		CARDIO:				
	SET 1		SET 2		SET 3		SET 4	
EXERCISE	WT.	REP	WT.	REP	WT.	REP	WT.	REP

DATE:		WT.		CARDIO:				
	SET 1		SET 2		SET 3		SET 4	
EXERCISE	WT.	REP	WT.	REP	WT.	REP	WT.	REP

DATE:		WT.		CARDIO:				
	SET 1		SET 2		SET 3		SET 4	
EXERCISE	WT.	REP	WT.	REP	WT.	REP	WT.	REP

WEEK 2

DATE:	WEIGHT:
HOW DO YOU FEEL?	
IF YOU CAN MEASURE IT, YOU CAN IMPROVE IT	

GOALS

1.
2.
3.

DATE:		WT.		CARDIO:			
	SET 1		SET 2		SET 3		SET 4	
EXERCISE	WT.	REP	WT.	REP	WT.	REP	WT.	REP

DATE:	WT.		CARDIO:					
	SET 1		SET 2		SET 3		SET 4	
EXERCISE	WT.	REP	WT.	REP	WT.	REP	WT.	REP

DATE:	WT.		CARDIO:					
	SET 1		SET 2		SET 3		SET 4	
EXERCISE	WT.	REP	WT.	REP	WT.	REP	WT.	REP

DATE:	WT.		CARDIO:					
	SET 1		SET 2		SET 3		SET 4	
EXERCISE	WT.	REP	WT.	REP	WT.	REP	WT.	REP

DATE:	WT.		CARDIO:					
	SET 1		SET 2		SET 3		SET 4	
EXERCISE	WT.	REP	WT.	REP	WT.	REP	WT.	REP

DATE:		WT.		CARDIO:				
	SET 1		SET 2		SET 3		SET 4	
EXERCISE	WT.	REP	WT.	REP	WT.	REP	WT.	REP

DATE:		WT.		CARDIO:				
	SET 1		SET 2		SET 3		SET 4	
EXERCISE	WT.	REP	WT.	REP	WT.	REP	WT.	REP

WEEK 3

DATE:	WEIGHT:

HOW DO YOU FEEL?

IF YOU CAN MEASURE IT, YOU CAN IMPROVE IT

GOALS

1.
2.
3.

DATE:		WT.		CARDIO:				
	SET 1		SET 2		SET 3		SET 4	
EXERCISE	WT.	REP	WT.	REP	WT.	REP	WT.	REP

DATE:		WT.		CARDIO:				
	SET 1		SET 2		SET 3		SET 4	
EXERCISE	WT.	REP	WT.	REP	WT.	REP	WT.	REP

DATE:		WT.		CARDIO:				
	SET 1		SET 2		SET 3		SET 4	
EXERCISE	WT.	REP	WT.	REP	WT.	REP	WT.	REP

Date:		Wt.		Cardio:				
	Set 1		Set 2		Set 3		Set 4	
Exercise	Wt.	Rep	Wt.	Rep	Wt.	Rep	Wt.	Rep

Date:		Wt.		Cardio:				
	Set 1		Set 2		Set 3		Set 4	
Exercise	Wt.	Rep	Wt.	Rep	Wt.	Rep	Wt.	Rep

DATE:		WT.		CARDIO:				
	SET 1		SET 2		SET 3		SET 4	
EXERCISE	WT.	REP	WT.	REP	WT.	REP	WT.	REP

DATE:		WT.		CARDIO:				
	SET 1		SET 2		SET 3		SET 4	
EXERCISE	WT.	REP	WT.	REP	WT.	REP	WT.	REP

WEEK 4

DATE:	WEIGHT:

HOW DO YOU FEEL?

IF YOU CAN MEASURE IT, YOU CAN IMPROVE IT

GOALS

1.
2.
3.

DATE:		WT.		CARDIO:				
	SET 1		SET 2		SET 3		SET 4	
EXERCISE	WT.	REP	WT.	REP	WT.	REP	WT.	REP

DATE:		WT.		CARDIO:				
	SET 1		SET 2		SET 3		SET 4	
EXERCISE	WT.	REP	WT.	REP	WT.	REP	WT.	REP

DATE:		WT.		CARDIO:				
	SET 1		SET 2		SET 3		SET 4	
EXERCISE	WT.	REP	WT.	REP	WT.	REP	WT.	REP

DATE:		WT.		CARDIO:			
	SET 1		SET 2		SET 3		SET 4	
EXERCISE	WT.	REP	WT.	REP	WT.	REP	WT.	REP

DATE:		WT.		CARDIO:			
	SET 1		SET 2		SET 3		SET 4	
EXERCISE	WT.	REP	WT.	REP	WT.	REP	WT.	REP

DATE:		WT.		CARDIO:				
	SET 1		SET 2		SET 3		SET 4	
EXERCISE	WT.	REP	WT.	REP	WT.	REP	WT.	REP

DATE:		WT.		CARDIO:				
	SET 1		SET 2		SET 3		SET 4	
EXERCISE	WT.	REP	WT.	REP	WT.	REP	WT.	REP

Week 5

Date:	Weight:
How do you feel?	
If you can measure it, you can improve it	

Goals

1.
2.
3.

Date:		Wt.		Cardio:			
	Set 1		Set 2		Set 3		Set 4	
Exercise	Wt.	Rep	Wt.	Rep	Wt.	Rep	Wt.	Rep

DATE:		WT.		CARDIO:				
	SET 1		SET 2		SET 3		SET 4	
EXERCISE	WT.	REP	WT.	REP	WT.	REP	WT.	REP

DATE:		WT.		CARDIO:				
	SET 1		SET 2		SET 3		SET 4	
EXERCISE	WT.	REP	WT.	REP	WT.	REP	WT.	REP

DATE:		WT.		CARDIO:				
	SET 1		SET 2		SET 3		SET 4	
EXERCISE	WT.	REP	WT.	REP	WT.	REP	WT.	REP

DATE:		WT.		CARDIO:				
	SET 1		SET 2		SET 3		SET 4	
EXERCISE	WT.	REP	WT.	REP	WT.	REP	WT.	REP

DATE:		WT.		CARDIO:				
	SET 1		SET 2		SET 3		SET 4	
EXERCISE	WT.	REP	WT.	REP	WT.	REP	WT.	REP

DATE:		WT.		CARDIO:				
	SET 1		SET 2		SET 3		SET 4	
EXERCISE	WT.	REP	WT.	REP	WT.	REP	WT.	REP

WEEK 6

DATE:	WEIGHT:

HOW DO YOU FEEL?

IF YOU CAN MEASURE IT, YOU CAN IMPROVE IT

GOALS

1.
2.
3.

DATE:		WT.		CARDIO:				
	SET 1		SET 2		SET 3		SET 4	
EXERCISE	WT.	REP	WT.	REP	WT.	REP	WT.	REP

DATE:		WT.		CARDIO:				
	SET 1		SET 2		SET 3		SET 4	
EXERCISE	WT.	REP	WT.	REP	WT.	REP	WT.	REP

DATE:		WT.		CARDIO:				
	SET 1		SET 2		SET 3		SET 4	
EXERCISE	WT.	REP	WT.	REP	WT.	REP	WT.	REP

DATE:		WT.		CARDIO:				
	SET 1		SET 2		SET 3		SET 4	
EXERCISE	WT.	REP	WT.	REP	WT.	REP	WT.	REP

DATE:		WT.		CARDIO:				
	SET 1		SET 2		SET 3		SET 4	
EXERCISE	WT.	REP	WT.	REP	WT.	REP	WT.	REP

DATE:		WT.		CARDIO:				
	SET 1		SET 2		SET 3		SET 4	
EXERCISE	WT.	REP	WT.	REP	WT.	REP	WT.	REP

DATE:		WT.		CARDIO:				
	SET 1		SET 2		SET 3		SET 4	
EXERCISE	WT.	REP	WT.	REP	WT.	REP	WT.	REP

WEEK 7	
DATE:	WEIGHT:
HOW DO YOU FEEL?	
IF YOU CAN MEASURE IT, YOU CAN IMPROVE IT	
GOALS	

1.
2.
3.

DATE:		WT.		CARDIO:				
	SET 1		SET 2		SET 3		SET 4	
EXERCISE	WT.	REP	WT.	REP	WT.	REP	WT.	REP

DATE:		WT.		CARDIO:				
	SET 1		SET 2		SET 3		SET 4	
EXERCISE	WT.	REP	WT.	REP	WT.	REP	WT.	REP

DATE:		WT.		CARDIO:				
	SET 1		SET 2		SET 3		SET 4	
EXERCISE	WT.	REP	WT.	REP	WT.	REP	WT.	REP

Date:		Wt.		Cardio:				
	Set 1		Set 2		Set 3		Set 4	
Exercise	Wt.	Rep	Wt.	Rep	Wt.	Rep	Wt.	Rep

Date:		Wt.		Cardio:				
	Set 1		Set 2		Set 3		Set 4	
Exercise	Wt.	Rep	Wt.	Rep	Wt.	Rep	Wt.	Rep

DATE:		WT.		CARDIO:				
	SET 1		SET 2		SET 3		SET 4	
EXERCISE	WT.	REP	WT.	REP	WT.	REP	WT.	REP

DATE:		WT.		CARDIO:				
	SET 1		SET 2		SET 3		SET 4	
EXERCISE	WT.	REP	WT.	REP	WT.	REP	WT.	REP

WEEK 8

DATE:	WEIGHT:
HOW DO YOU FEEL?	
IF YOU CAN MEASURE IT, YOU CAN IMPROVE IT	

GOALS

1.
2.
3.

DATE:	WT.		CARDIO:					
	SET 1		SET 2		SET 3		SET 4	
EXERCISE	WT.	REP	WT.	REP	WT.	REP	WT.	REP

Date:		Wt.		Cardio:			
	Set 1		Set 2		Set 3		Set 4	
Exercise	Wt.	Rep	Wt.	Rep	Wt.	Rep	Wt.	Rep

Date:		Wt.		Cardio:			
	Set 1		Set 2		Set 3		Set 4	
Exercise	Wt.	Rep	Wt.	Rep	Wt.	Rep	Wt.	Rep

Date:		Wt.		Cardio:				
	Set 1		Set 2		Set 3		Set 4	
Exercise	Wt.	Rep	Wt.	Rep	Wt.	Rep	Wt.	Rep

Date:		Wt.		Cardio:				
	Set 1		Set 2		Set 3		Set 4	
Exercise	Wt.	Rep	Wt.	Rep	Wt.	Rep	Wt.	Rep

DATE:		WT.		CARDIO:				
	SET 1		SET 2		SET 3		SET 4	
EXERCISE	WT.	REP	WT.	REP	WT.	REP	WT.	REP

DATE:		WT.		CARDIO:				
	SET 1		SET 2		SET 3		SET 4	
EXERCISE	WT.	REP	WT.	REP	WT.	REP	WT.	REP

WEEK 9

DATE:	WEIGHT:
HOW DO YOU FEEL?	
IF YOU CAN MEASURE IT, YOU CAN IMPROVE IT	

GOALS

1.
2.
3.

DATE:		WT.		CARDIO:				
	SET 1		SET 2		SET 3		SET 4	
EXERCISE	WT.	REP	WT.	REP	WT.	REP	WT.	REP

DATE:		WT.		CARDIO:				
	SET 1		SET 2		SET 3		SET 4	
EXERCISE	WT.	REP	WT.	REP	WT.	REP	WT.	REP

DATE:		WT.		CARDIO:				
	SET 1		SET 2		SET 3		SET 4	
EXERCISE	WT.	REP	WT.	REP	WT.	REP	WT.	REP

DATE:		WT.		CARDIO:				
	SET 1		SET 2		SET 3		SET 4	
EXERCISE	WT.	REP	WT.	REP	WT.	REP	WT.	REP

DATE:		WT.		CARDIO:				
	SET 1		SET 2		SET 3		SET 4	
EXERCISE	WT.	REP	WT.	REP	WT.	REP	WT.	REP

DATE:		WT.		CARDIO:				
	SET 1		SET 2		SET 3		SET 4	
EXERCISE	WT.	REP	WT.	REP	WT.	REP	WT.	REP

DATE:		WT.		CARDIO:				
	SET 1		SET 2		SET 3		SET 4	
EXERCISE	WT.	REP	WT.	REP	WT.	REP	WT.	REP

WEEK 10

DATE:	WEIGHT:

HOW DO YOU FEEL?

IF YOU CAN MEASURE IT, YOU CAN IMPROVE IT

GOALS

1.
2.
3.

DATE:		WT.		CARDIO:				
	SET 1		SET 2		SET 3		SET 4	
EXERCISE	WT.	REP	WT.	REP	WT.	REP	WT.	REP

Date:		Wt.		Cardio:				
	Set 1		Set 2		Set 3		Set 4	
Exercise	Wt.	Rep	Wt.	Rep	Wt.	Rep	Wt.	Rep

Date:		Wt.		Cardio:				
	Set 1		Set 2		Set 3		Set 4	
Exercise	Wt.	Rep	Wt.	Rep	Wt.	Rep	Wt.	Rep

DATE:		WT.		CARDIO:				
	SET 1		SET 2		SET 3		SET 4	
EXERCISE	WT.	REP	WT.	REP	WT.	REP	WT.	REP

DATE:		WT.		CARDIO:				
	SET 1		SET 2		SET 3		SET 4	
EXERCISE	WT.	REP	WT.	REP	WT.	REP	WT.	REP

Date:		Wt.		Cardio:				
	Set 1		Set 2		Set 3		Set 4	
Exercise	Wt.	Rep	Wt.	Rep	Wt.	Rep	Wt.	Rep

Date:		Wt.		Cardio:				
	Set 1		Set 2		Set 3		Set 4	
Exercise	Wt.	Rep	Wt.	Rep	Wt.	Rep	Wt.	Rep

WEEK 11	
DATE:	WEIGHT:
HOW DO YOU FEEL?	
IF YOU CAN MEASURE IT, YOU CAN IMPROVE IT	
GOALS	
1.	
2.	
3.	

DATE:		WT.		CARDIO:				
	SET 1		SET 2		SET 3		SET 4	
EXERCISE	WT.	REP	WT.	REP	WT.	REP	WT.	REP

DATE:		WT.		CARDIO:				
	SET 1		SET 2		SET 3		SET 4	
EXERCISE	WT.	REP	WT.	REP	WT.	REP	WT.	REP

DATE:		WT.		CARDIO:				
	SET 1		SET 2		SET 3		SET 4	
EXERCISE	WT.	REP	WT.	REP	WT.	REP	WT.	REP

DATE:		WT.		CARDIO:				
	SET 1		SET 2		SET 3		SET 4	
EXERCISE	WT.	REP	WT.	REP	WT.	REP	WT.	REP

DATE:		WT.		CARDIO:				
	SET 1		SET 2		SET 3		SET 4	
EXERCISE	WT.	REP	WT.	REP	WT.	REP	WT.	REP

DATE:		WT.		CARDIO:				
	SET 1		SET 2		SET 3		SET 4	
EXERCISE	WT.	REP	WT.	REP	WT.	REP	WT.	REP

DATE:		WT.		CARDIO:				
	SET 1		SET 2		SET 3		SET 4	
EXERCISE	WT.	REP	WT.	REP	WT.	REP	WT.	REP

WEEK 12

DATE:	WEIGHT:

HOW DO YOU FEEL?

IF YOU CAN MEASURE IT, YOU CAN IMPROVE IT

GOALS

1.
2.
3.

DATE:		WT.		CARDIO:				
	SET 1		SET 2		SET 3		SET 4	
EXERCISE	WT.	REP	WT.	REP	WT.	REP	WT.	REP

Date:	WT.		Cardio:					
	Set 1		Set 2		Set 3		Set 4	
Exercise	Wt.	Rep	Wt.	Rep	Wt.	Rep	Wt.	Rep

Date:	WT.		Cardio:					
	Set 1		Set 2		Set 3		Set 4	
Exercise	Wt.	Rep	Wt.	Rep	Wt.	Rep	Wt.	Rep

DATE:		WT.		CARDIO:				
	SET 1		SET 2		SET 3		SET 4	
EXERCISE	WT.	REP	WT.	REP	WT.	REP	WT.	REP

DATE:		WT.		CARDIO:				
	SET 1		SET 2		SET 3		SET 4	
EXERCISE	WT.	REP	WT.	REP	WT.	REP	WT.	REP

DATE:	WT.		CARDIO:					
	SET 1		SET 2		SET 3		SET 4	
EXERCISE	WT.	REP	WT.	REP	WT.	REP	WT.	REP

DATE:	WT.		CARDIO:					
	SET 1		SET 2		SET 3		SET 4	
EXERCISE	WT.	REP	WT.	REP	WT.	REP	WT.	REP

WEEK 13

DATE:	WEIGHT:

HOW DO YOU FEEL?

IF YOU CAN MEASURE IT, YOU CAN IMPROVE IT

GOALS

1.
2.
3.

DATE:		WT.		CARDIO:				
	SET 1		SET 2		SET 3		SET 4	
EXERCISE	WT.	REP	WT.	REP	WT.	REP	WT.	REP

DATE:		WT.		CARDIO:				
	SET 1		SET 2		SET 3		SET 4	
EXERCISE	WT.	REP	WT.	REP	WT.	REP	WT.	REP

DATE:		WT.		CARDIO:				
	SET 1		SET 2		SET 3		SET 4	
EXERCISE	WT.	REP	WT.	REP	WT.	REP	WT.	REP

DATE:		WT.		CARDIO:				
	SET 1		SET 2		SET 3		SET 4	
EXERCISE	WT.	REP	WT.	REP	WT.	REP	WT.	REP

DATE:		WT.		CARDIO:				
	SET 1		SET 2		SET 3		SET 4	
EXERCISE	WT.	REP	WT.	REP	WT.	REP	WT.	REP

Date:		Wt.		Cardio:			
	Set 1		Set 2		Set 3		Set 4	
Exercise	Wt.	Rep	Wt.	Rep	Wt.	Rep	Wt.	Rep

Date:		Wt.		Cardio:			
	Set 1		Set 2		Set 3		Set 4	
Exercise	Wt.	Rep	Wt.	Rep	Wt.	Rep	Wt.	Rep

WEEK 14

DATE:	WEIGHT:

HOW DO YOU FEEL?

IF YOU CAN MEASURE IT, YOU CAN IMPROVE IT

GOALS

1.
2.
3.

DATE:		WT.		CARDIO:				
	SET 1		SET 2		SET 3		SET 4	
EXERCISE	WT.	REP	WT.	REP	WT.	REP	WT.	REP

Date:		Wt.		Cardio:				
	Set 1		Set 2		Set 3		Set 4	
Exercise	Wt.	Rep	Wt.	Rep	Wt.	Rep	Wt.	Rep

Date:		Wt.		Cardio:				
	Set 1		Set 2		Set 3		Set 4	
Exercise	Wt.	Rep	Wt.	Rep	Wt.	Rep	Wt.	Rep

Date:		Wt.		Cardio:				
	Set 1		Set 2		Set 3		Set 4	
Exercise	Wt.	Rep	Wt.	Rep	Wt.	Rep	Wt.	Rep

Date:		Wt.		Cardio:				
	Set 1		Set 2		Set 3		Set 4	
Exercise	Wt.	Rep	Wt.	Rep	Wt.	Rep	Wt.	Rep

Date:		Wt.		Cardio:				
	Set 1		Set 2		Set 3		Set 4	
Exercise	Wt.	Rep	Wt.	Rep	Wt.	Rep	Wt.	Rep

Date:		Wt.		Cardio:				
	Set 1		Set 2		Set 3		Set 4	
Exercise	Wt.	Rep	Wt.	Rep	Wt.	Rep	Wt.	Rep

WEEK 15

DATE:	WEIGHT:

HOW DO YOU FEEL?

IF YOU CAN MEASURE IT, YOU CAN IMPROVE IT

GOALS

1.
2.
3.

DATE:		WT.		CARDIO:				
	SET 1		SET 2		SET 3		SET 4	
EXERCISE	WT.	REP	WT.	REP	WT.	REP	WT.	REP

DATE:		WT.		CARDIO:				
	SET 1		SET 2		SET 3		SET 4	
EXERCISE	WT.	REP	WT.	REP	WT.	REP	WT.	REP

DATE:		WT.		CARDIO:				
	SET 1		SET 2		SET 3		SET 4	
EXERCISE	WT.	REP	WT.	REP	WT.	REP	WT.	REP

Date:		Wt.		Cardio:				
	Set 1		Set 2		Set 3		Set 4	
Exercise	Wt.	Rep	Wt.	Rep	Wt.	Rep	Wt.	Rep

Date:		Wt.		Cardio:				
	Set 1		Set 2		Set 3		Set 4	
Exercise	Wt.	Rep	Wt.	Rep	Wt.	Rep	Wt.	Rep

DATE:		WT.		CARDIO:				
	SET 1		SET 2		SET 3		SET 4	
EXERCISE	WT.	REP	WT.	REP	WT.	REP	WT.	REP

DATE:		WT.		CARDIO:				
	SET 1		SET 2		SET 3		SET 4	
EXERCISE	WT.	REP	WT.	REP	WT.	REP	WT.	REP

WEEK 16

DATE:	WEIGHT:
HOW DO YOU FEEL?	
IF YOU CAN MEASURE IT, YOU CAN IMPROVE IT	

GOALS

1.
2.
3.

DATE:		WT.		CARDIO:				
	SET 1		SET 2		SET 3		SET 4	
EXERCISE	WT.	REP	WT.	REP	WT.	REP	WT.	REP

Date:		Wt.		Cardio:				
	Set 1		Set 2		Set 3		Set 4	
Exercise	Wt.	Rep	Wt.	Rep	Wt.	Rep	Wt.	Rep

Date:		Wt.		Cardio:				
	Set 1		Set 2		Set 3		Set 4	
Exercise	Wt.	Rep	Wt.	Rep	Wt.	Rep	Wt.	Rep

DATE:		WT.		CARDIO:			
	SET 1		SET 2		SET 3		SET 4	
EXERCISE	WT.	REP	WT.	REP	WT.	REP	WT.	REP

DATE:		WT.		CARDIO:			
	SET 1		SET 2		SET 3		SET 4	
EXERCISE	WT.	REP	WT.	REP	WT.	REP	WT.	REP

DATE:		WT.		CARDIO:			
	SET 1		SET 2		SET 3		SET 4	
EXERCISE	WT.	REP	WT.	REP	WT.	REP	WT.	REP

DATE:		WT.		CARDIO:			
	SET 1		SET 2		SET 3		SET 4	
EXERCISE	WT.	REP	WT.	REP	WT.	REP	WT.	REP

Week 17

Date:	Weight:
How do you feel?	
If you can measure it, you can improve it	

Goals

1.
2.
3.

Date:		Wt.		Cardio:				
	Set 1		Set 2		Set 3		Set 4	
Exercise	Wt.	Rep	Wt.	Rep	Wt.	Rep	Wt.	Rep

DATE:		WT.		CARDIO:				
	SET 1		SET 2		SET 3		SET 4	
EXERCISE	WT.	REP	WT.	REP	WT.	REP	WT.	REP

DATE:		WT.		CARDIO:				
	SET 1		SET 2		SET 3		SET 4	
EXERCISE	WT.	REP	WT.	REP	WT.	REP	WT.	REP

Date:		Wt.		Cardio:				
	Set 1		Set 2		Set 3		Set 4	
Exercise	Wt.	Rep	Wt.	Rep	Wt.	Rep	Wt.	Rep

Date:		Wt.		Cardio:				
	Set 1		Set 2		Set 3		Set 4	
Exercise	Wt.	Rep	Wt.	Rep	Wt.	Rep	Wt.	Rep

DATE:		WT.		CARDIO:				
	SET 1		SET 2		SET 3		SET 4	
EXERCISE	WT.	REP	WT.	REP	WT.	REP	WT.	REP

DATE:		WT.		CARDIO:				
	SET 1		SET 2		SET 3		SET 4	
EXERCISE	WT.	REP	WT.	REP	WT.	REP	WT.	REP

WEEK 18

DATE:	WEIGHT:

HOW DO YOU FEEL?

IF YOU CAN MEASURE IT, YOU CAN IMPROVE IT

GOALS

1.
2.
3.

DATE:		WT.		CARDIO:				
	SET 1		SET 2		SET 3		SET 4	
EXERCISE	WT.	REP	WT.	REP	WT.	REP	WT.	REP

DATE:		WT.		CARDIO:				
	SET 1		SET 2		SET 3		SET 4	
EXERCISE	WT.	REP	WT.	REP	WT.	REP	WT.	REP

DATE:		WT.		CARDIO:				
	SET 1		SET 2		SET 3		SET 4	
EXERCISE	WT.	REP	WT.	REP	WT.	REP	WT.	REP

DATE:		WT.		CARDIO:				
	SET 1		SET 2		SET 3		SET 4	
EXERCISE	WT.	REP	WT.	REP	WT.	REP	WT.	REP

DATE:		WT.		CARDIO:				
	SET 1		SET 2		SET 3		SET 4	
EXERCISE	WT.	REP	WT.	REP	WT.	REP	WT.	REP

DATE:		WT.		CARDIO:				
	SET 1		SET 2		SET 3		SET 4	
EXERCISE	WT.	REP	WT.	REP	WT.	REP	WT.	REP

DATE:		WT.		CARDIO:				
	SET 1		SET 2		SET 3		SET 4	
EXERCISE	WT.	REP	WT.	REP	WT.	REP	WT.	REP

WEEK 19

DATE:	WEIGHT:

HOW DO YOU FEEL?

IF YOU CAN MEASURE IT, YOU CAN IMPROVE IT

GOALS

1.
2.
3.

DATE:		WT.		CARDIO:				
	SET 1		SET 2		SET 3		SET 4	
EXERCISE	WT.	REP	WT.	REP	WT.	REP	WT.	REP

DATE:		WT.		CARDIO:				
	SET 1		SET 2		SET 3		SET 4	
EXERCISE	WT.	REP	WT.	REP	WT.	REP	WT.	REP

DATE:		WT.		CARDIO:				
	SET 1		SET 2		SET 3		SET 4	
EXERCISE	WT.	REP	WT.	REP	WT.	REP	WT.	REP

DATE:		WT.		CARDIO:			
	SET 1		SET 2		SET 3		SET 4	
EXERCISE	WT.	REP	WT.	REP	WT.	REP	WT.	REP

DATE:		WT.		CARDIO:			
	SET 1		SET 2		SET 3		SET 4	
EXERCISE	WT.	REP	WT.	REP	WT.	REP	WT.	REP

DATE:		WT.		CARDIO:				
	SET 1		SET 2		SET 3		SET 4	
EXERCISE	WT.	REP	WT.	REP	WT.	REP	WT.	REP

DATE:		WT.		CARDIO:				
	SET 1		SET 2		SET 3		SET 4	
EXERCISE	WT.	REP	WT.	REP	WT.	REP	WT.	REP

WEEK 20

DATE:	WEIGHT:

HOW DO YOU FEEL?

IF YOU CAN MEASURE IT, YOU CAN IMPROVE IT

GOALS

1.
2.
3.

DATE:		WT.		CARDIO:				
	SET 1		SET 2		SET 3		SET 4	
EXERCISE	WT.	REP	WT.	REP	WT.	REP	WT.	REP

DATE:		WT.		CARDIO:				
	SET 1		SET 2		SET 3		SET 4	
EXERCISE	WT.	REP	WT.	REP	WT.	REP	WT.	REP

DATE:		WT.		CARDIO:				
	SET 1		SET 2		SET 3		SET 4	
EXERCISE	WT.	REP	WT.	REP	WT.	REP	WT.	REP

DATE:		WT.		CARDIO:				
	SET 1		SET 2		SET 3		SET 4	
EXERCISE	WT.	REP	WT.	REP	WT.	REP	WT.	REP

DATE:		WT.		CARDIO:				
	SET 1		SET 2		SET 3		SET 4	
EXERCISE	WT.	REP	WT.	REP	WT.	REP	WT.	REP

Date:		Wt.		Cardio:				
	Set 1		Set 2		Set 3		Set 4	
Exercise	Wt.	Rep	Wt.	Rep	Wt.	Rep	Wt.	Rep

Date:		Wt.		Cardio:				
	Set 1		Set 2		Set 3		Set 4	
Exercise	Wt.	Rep	Wt.	Rep	Wt.	Rep	Wt.	Rep

WEEK 21

DATE:	WEIGHT:
HOW DO YOU FEEL?	
IF YOU CAN MEASURE IT, YOU CAN IMPROVE IT	

GOALS

1.
2.
3.

DATE:	WT.		CARDIO:					
	SET 1		SET 2		SET 3		SET 4	
EXERCISE	WT.	REP	WT.	REP	WT.	REP	WT.	REP

Date:		Wt.		Cardio:				
	Set 1		Set 2		Set 3		Set 4	
Exercise	Wt.	Rep	Wt.	Rep	Wt.	Rep	Wt.	Rep

Date:		Wt.		Cardio:				
	Set 1		Set 2		Set 3		Set 4	
Exercise	Wt.	Rep	Wt.	Rep	Wt.	Rep	Wt.	Rep

DATE:		WT.		CARDIO:				
	SET 1		SET 2		SET 3		SET 4	
EXERCISE	WT.	REP	WT.	REP	WT.	REP	WT.	REP

DATE:		WT.		CARDIO:				
	SET 1		SET 2		SET 3		SET 4	
EXERCISE	WT.	REP	WT.	REP	WT.	REP	WT.	REP

Date:		Wt.		Cardio:				
	Set 1		Set 2		Set 3		Set 4	
Exercise	Wt.	Rep	Wt.	Rep	Wt.	Rep	Wt.	Rep

Date:		Wt.		Cardio:				
	Set 1		Set 2		Set 3		Set 4	
Exercise	Wt.	Rep	Wt.	Rep	Wt.	Rep	Wt.	Rep

WEEK 22	
DATE:	WEIGHT:
HOW DO YOU FEEL?	
IF YOU CAN MEASURE IT, YOU CAN IMPROVE IT	
GOALS	
1.	
2.	
3.	

DATE:		WT.		CARDIO:				
	SET 1		SET 2		SET 3		SET 4	
EXERCISE	WT.	REP	WT.	REP	WT.	REP	WT.	REP

DATE:		WT.		CARDIO:				
	SET 1		SET 2		SET 3		SET 4	
EXERCISE	WT.	REP	WT.	REP	WT.	REP	WT.	REP

DATE:		WT.		CARDIO:				
	SET 1		SET 2		SET 3		SET 4	
EXERCISE	WT.	REP	WT.	REP	WT.	REP	WT.	REP

DATE:		WT.		CARDIO:				
	SET 1		SET 2		SET 3		SET 4	
EXERCISE	WT.	REP	WT.	REP	WT.	REP	WT.	REP

DATE:		WT.		CARDIO:				
	SET 1		SET 2		SET 3		SET 4	
EXERCISE	WT.	REP	WT.	REP	WT.	REP	WT.	REP

DATE:		WT.		CARDIO:				
	SET 1		SET 2		SET 3		SET 4	
EXERCISE	WT.	REP	WT.	REP	WT.	REP	WT.	REP

DATE:		WT.		CARDIO:				
	SET 1		SET 2		SET 3		SET 4	
EXERCISE	WT.	REP	WT.	REP	WT.	REP	WT.	REP

WEEK 23

DATE:	WEIGHT:
HOW DO YOU FEEL?	
IF YOU CAN MEASURE IT, YOU CAN IMPROVE IT	

GOALS

1.
2.
3.

DATE:		WT.		CARDIO:			
	SET 1		SET 2		SET 3		SET 4	
EXERCISE	WT.	REP	WT.	REP	WT.	REP	WT.	REP

DATE:		WT.		CARDIO:				
	SET 1		SET 2		SET 3		SET 4	
EXERCISE	WT.	REP	WT.	REP	WT.	REP	WT.	REP

DATE:		WT.		CARDIO:				
	SET 1		SET 2		SET 3		SET 4	
EXERCISE	WT.	REP	WT.	REP	WT.	REP	WT.	REP

DATE:		WT.		CARDIO:				
	SET 1		SET 2		SET 3		SET 4	
EXERCISE	WT.	REP	WT.	REP	WT.	REP	WT.	REP

DATE:		WT.		CARDIO:				
	SET 1		SET 2		SET 3		SET 4	
EXERCISE	WT.	REP	WT.	REP	WT.	REP	WT.	REP

DATE:		WT.		CARDIO:				
	SET 1		SET 2		SET 3		SET 4	
EXERCISE	WT.	REP	WT.	REP	WT.	REP	WT.	REP

DATE:		WT.		CARDIO:				
	SET 1		SET 2		SET 3		SET 4	
EXERCISE	WT.	REP	WT.	REP	WT.	REP	WT.	REP

Week 24

Date:	Weight:

How do you feel?

If you can measure it, you can improve it

Goals

1.
2.
3.

Date:	WT.		Cardio:					
	Set 1		Set 2		Set 3		Set 4	
Exercise	WT.	Rep	WT.	Rep	WT.	Rep	WT.	Rep

DATE:		WT.		CARDIO:				
	SET 1		SET 2		SET 3		SET 4	
EXERCISE	WT.	REP	WT.	REP	WT.	REP	WT.	REP

DATE:		WT.		CARDIO:				
	SET 1		SET 2		SET 3		SET 4	
EXERCISE	WT.	REP	WT.	REP	WT.	REP	WT.	REP

Date:		Wt.		Cardio:				
	Set 1		Set 2		Set 3		Set 4	
Exercise	Wt.	Rep	Wt.	Rep	Wt.	Rep	Wt.	Rep

Date:		Wt.		Cardio:				
	Set 1		Set 2		Set 3		Set 4	
Exercise	Wt.	Rep	Wt.	Rep	Wt.	Rep	Wt.	Rep

DATE:		WT.		CARDIO:				
	SET 1		SET 2		SET 3		SET 4	
EXERCISE	WT.	REP	WT.	REP	WT.	REP	WT.	REP

DATE:		WT.		CARDIO:				
	SET 1		SET 2		SET 3		SET 4	
EXERCISE	WT.	REP	WT.	REP	WT.	REP	WT.	REP

Week 25

Date:		Weight:
How do you feel?		
If you can measure it, you can improve it		

Goals

1.
2.
3.

Date:		Wt.		Cardio:				
	Set 1		Set 2		Set 3		Set 4	
Exercise	Wt.	Rep	Wt.	Rep	Wt.	Rep	Wt.	Rep

DATE:		WT.		CARDIO:				
	SET 1		SET 2		SET 3		SET 4	
EXERCISE	WT.	REP	WT.	REP	WT.	REP	WT.	REP

DATE:		WT.		CARDIO:				
	SET 1		SET 2		SET 3		SET 4	
EXERCISE	WT.	REP	WT.	REP	WT.	REP	WT.	REP

DATE:		WT.		CARDIO:				
	SET 1		SET 2		SET 3		SET 4	
EXERCISE	WT.	REP	WT.	REP	WT.	REP	WT.	REP

DATE:		WT.		CARDIO:				
	SET 1		SET 2		SET 3		SET 4	
EXERCISE	WT.	REP	WT.	REP	WT.	REP	WT.	REP

Date:		WT.		Cardio:			
	Set 1		Set 2		Set 3		Set 4	
Exercise	Wt.	Rep	Wt.	Rep	Wt.	Rep	Wt.	Rep

Date:		WT.		Cardio:			
	Set 1		Set 2		Set 3		Set 4	
Exercise	Wt.	Rep	Wt.	Rep	Wt.	Rep	Wt.	Rep

WEEK 26

DATE:	WEIGHT:
HOW DO YOU FEEL?	
IF YOU CAN MEASURE IT, YOU CAN IMPROVE IT	

GOALS

1.
2.
3.

DATE:	WT.		CARDIO:					
	SET 1		SET 2		SET 3		SET 4	
EXERCISE	WT.	REP	WT.	REP	WT.	REP	WT.	REP

DATE:		WT.		CARDIO:				
	SET 1		SET 2		SET 3		SET 4	
EXERCISE	WT.	REP	WT.	REP	WT.	REP	WT.	REP

DATE:		WT.		CARDIO:				
	SET 1		SET 2		SET 3		SET 4	
EXERCISE	WT.	REP	WT.	REP	WT.	REP	WT.	REP

Date:		Wt.		Cardio:				
	Set 1		Set 2		Set 3		Set 4	
Exercise	Wt.	Rep	Wt.	Rep	Wt.	Rep	Wt.	Rep

Date:		Wt.		Cardio:				
	Set 1		Set 2		Set 3		Set 4	
Exercise	Wt.	Rep	Wt.	Rep	Wt.	Rep	Wt.	Rep

Date:		Wt.		Cardio:				
	Set 1		Set 2		Set 3		Set 4	
Exercise	Wt.	Rep	Wt.	Rep	Wt.	Rep	Wt.	Rep

Date:		Wt.		Cardio:				
	Set 1		Set 2		Set 3		Set 4	
Exercise	Wt.	Rep	Wt.	Rep	Wt.	Rep	Wt.	Rep

www.ingramcontent.com/pod-product-compliance
Lightning Source LLC
Chambersburg PA
CBHW060420290526
45791CB00002B/831